Table of Contents

A Beginner's Guide to the Keto Diet

A Tasty, Easy, and Rewarding Diet Plan to Help With Weight Loss and Maintain Your Desired Weight Goal

Amadeus Sorensen

Keto-Friendly Foods

   Vegetables

   Fruits

   Ground Meat

   Lunch and Deli Meats

   Meat and Poultry

   Seafood

   Dairy

   Fats and Oils

   Nuts and Seeds

   Keto-Friendly Drink Options

   Sauces and Dressings

   Canned Food

   Herbs and Spices

   Nut and Seed Butters

   Baking Ingredients

   Keto-Friendly Alcohol

   Vegetarian

   Keto Sweeteners

Non-Keto-Friendly Foods

   Grains

   Starches

   Flours

   Oils From Processed Vegetables and Trans Fats

Introduction

Consider *A Beginner's Guide to the Keto Diet* an introduction to food and wellness that offers a different and practical approach to nutrition. Throughout this book, I will discuss the fundamental value of a low-carb protein-dense, and high-fat diet—also known as the "keto diet"—in promoting good nutrition and treating various health conditions and ailments. Most fad dietary guidelines adopted by the public aren't supported by evidence or effective for the average person. *A Beginner's Guide to the Keto Diet* explains in plain English the latest research by highlighting the health benefits of ketones, including weight loss.

I'm glad you made this important decision. You are joining a growing number of individuals who have chosen to live healthier lives and are now reaping the benefits. Having a keto diet meal plan is crucial to achieving optimum results. Eating the right foods, eliminating the wrong ones, and meal planning is essential. Take advantage of the 7-day keto meal plan—the ideal way to start your keto journey. You can adhere to a strict diet or customize it to fit your needs. It's time to rethink your entire dietary philosophy and embrace this new way of living.

Chapter 1: What Is a Ketogenic Diet?

Ketogenic diets are characterized by high fat and low carbohydrate intake. Instead of carbohydrates, or 'carbs,' fat is burned for energy. Glucose is produced when carbohydrates are converted to sugar, which provides energy to the body and the brain (Mawer, 2020). In the event that you don't consume enough carbohydrates, your body will begin to burn fat. Your liver will burn the fat you consume and the fat you have stored in your body. The fat in your body is divided into two components: fatty acids and ketones. Ketones provide energy to your brain in place of glucose. Ketosis is a condition in which you have high levels of ketone bodies.

When I first learned about the 'keto' way of life, I was eager to learn more. After reading numerous books and academic articles as well as observing others yield positive and successful results, I applied the theory myself and I too was transformed!

The keto diet isn't about counting calories. Instead, the attention is on the fat, carbohydrate, and protein content of the meals and portion sizes you consume.

So what triggered the Keto Diet? Almost a century ago, Russell Wilder, a Mayo Clinic doctor, created the Ketogenic Diet in an attempt to treat epilepsy by mimicking starvation in the body (Licquia, 2017). People who suffer from epilepsy and similar diseases reported a reduction in symptoms following a keto diet. Greco-Roman physicians practiced a similar diet but starved their patients. Ketogenic diets provide an effortless way to induce fasting without starving oneself. To be frank, however, no one knows why the diet benefits people suffering from seizures, developmental disorders, and other illnesses.

A ketogenic diet usually is composed of 60–75% fats, 15–30% protein, and 5–10% carbohydrates. Keto meals are typically high-fat, low-carb, and contain a moderate amount of protein. Examples of such meals include white fish, with a side of berries or broccoli, supplemented with a high-fat content food like cheese. On this diet, fats are primarily derived from ingredients used in cooking; these may include avocado oil, ghee, or olive oil, as well as rich condiments like sour cream.

Chapter 2: Advantages of the Keto Diet

Potentially Can Prevent Cancer

A study on whether a ketogenic diet might benefit cancer detection and management has recently begun. Human studies are few, although animal and laboratory experiments have examined the role that ketosis plays in cancer.

Animal Studies

These studies, along with those conducted on laboratory cancer cells, cannot accurately predict human responses, but they offer a glimpse into keto's cancer-fighting potential. The results of studies on animals indicate keto may possess cancer-fighting properties. In a review of studies published in 2017, 72% showed that a keto diet prevented cancer in animals. According to this study, a keto diet did not aggravate tumors (Eldridge, 2022). Cancer cells also appear to be affected by a keto diet. According to a study published in 2019, the keto diet suppresses cellular activity in ways that extend beyond reducing energy production. The reason, however, is unclear (Eldridge, 2022).

Human Studies

Studies on the keto diet practiced by cancer patients are limited, and nearly all are preventative. Some convincing proof comes from evidence of its effects on glioblastoma, the most prevalent and deadly form of brain cancer. A keto diet may also be helpful for other cancers, such as lung, colon, pancreatic, and prostate cancer.

Although studies on animals are helpful, human studies may differ in their outcomes and factors. A study on the effects of keto dieting in women with ovarian or uterine cancer was primarily concerned with its preventative aspects, but it also demonstrated promise in other areas. The diet did not adversely affect the well-being of the women and may have improved their physical performance, energy level, and appetite (Eldridge, 2022).

Keto and Metabolism

People frequently have questions about ketosis and metabolism. It is widely thought that a ketogenic diet can slow down metabolism or inhibit it. The ketogenic diet has been shown to have weight-loss benefits, yet some people believe it slows your metabolism over time, which is a legitimate concern since other diets do the same thing.

Any diet involving calorie restriction will lower metabolism. To stay in a deficit for more than three weeks, you need to be concerned about your metabolism regardless of whether you eat carbs or not. Therefore, this is not a keto diet issue. When you follow a keto diet, you can boost your metabolic rate or maintain its level, albeit at a higher rate than before. A person's basal metabolic rate (BMR) determines how many calories they burn each day, no matter how much they exercise. A person's BMR is directly related to their weight, meaning that larger individuals require more energy to maintain their weight.

Typically, when someone rapidly loses weight, their BMR decreases as a direct result of losing weight. Consequently, they will eventually be prone to putting on weight once they stop their diet and workout routine. Despite this, on the keto diet, your metabolic rate does not change as you shed pounds. Ketosis prevents muscle loss, which in turn keeps your metabolic rate in check. Regardless of your weight, the more muscle and less fat you have, the better your metabolism. This is because, at rest, muscle burns more calories than fat.

Keto and Hormonal Balance

Properly implementing a keto diet can assist women in regaining hormonal balance. It can reduce body fat, hot flashes, fatigue, low libido, osteoporosis, mood changes, and other unpleasant side effects linked with menopause, perimenopause, premenstrual syndrome, and other midlife conditions. Therefore, the keto diet is ideal for females experiencing hormonal fluctuations.

You need fat to survive on a keto diet. On a traditional keto diet, 75% of your diet should consist of healthy fats. Great sources of healthy fats include avocados, almonds, flaxseeds, coconut oil, ghee, olives and olive oil, and other fat-rich foods. These 'good' fats help regulate and keep hormone levels in check because of how fats assist in testosterone, progesterone, and estrogen production. We have been told for too long to avoid fat, so we cut out fat instead of carbohydrates. It was a bad move, and I believe the low-fat trend is responsible for hormone problems among women today.

A ketogenic diet limits carbs to 20–50 grams daily. It balances blood sugar levels by reducing the release of insulin in the body. Insulin regulates your sugar levels, and if your levels are too elevated and unbalanced, you may experience a drop in hormone levels. Ketogenic diets make your body more insulin responsive. Insulin is therefore properly controlled, kept in check, and metabolized effectively by your cells. The Annals of Internal Medicine published a study in 2005 showing that a ketogenic diet improved insulin sensitivity in people who were obese and diabetic by 75% (Boden et al., 2005).

Despite the lack of studies conducted across the broader population, the findings are encouraging. Insulin sensitivity makes metabolic transformations possible: You lose weight and become fit; you diminish your chances of developing heart disease and Alzheimer's; you're less likely to experience hot flashes or sweaty nights; you strengthen your bones and prevent bone loss and osteoporosis; you have fewer cravings; you look and feel more energetic.

Keto Diet and Brain Health

Scientists have discovered that fat can be a powerful nutrient for the brain, helping neurons burn glucose more effectively with age. Recent studies suggest that a keto diet may help Alzheimer's patients think better and decrease others' risk of developing the disease (Sullivan, 2021).

How does the keto diet affect the brain? It offers another source of fuel. Normally, the brain consumes glucose. Sugar is derived from carbohydrates, and the mitochondria, which power every living cell, converts it into energy. However, when carbs are scarce, or not present, the brain can resort to a backup fuel: ketones. Similar to glucose, which occurs as a result of carbohydrate breakdown, ketones are produced by fat digestion.

Fat is stored for future needs, or it can be burned as fuel. Fat can be burned by some tissues directly while others, such as neurons, cannot. Liver enzymes convert fat into ketones. Upon entering the bloodstream, they are carried to the brain, where they are used as energy. The long-term objective is not to put everyone on a ketogenic diet but to understand more about how fat consumption impacts the brain.

Chapter 3: How to Get Into Ketosis

The ketogenic diet is marked by the metabolic state of ketosis. In a standard diet, your body largely depends on sugar or, to be precise, glucose. Carbohydrates are the best way to acquire this type of energy because they're high in sugar and digest rapidly. However, fats and proteins can also produce glucose in a process known as gluconeogenesis, which is more gradual.

Limiting your carbohydrate consumption—under 50 grams daily—can significantly change how your body burns energy. In other words, if you don't have enough carbohydrates to produce glucose, your body will turn to fat as an alternate fuel source.

Regardless of your diet, even if you eat a lot of carbohydrates, your body burns fat for energy, primarily during sleep and when you aren't eating. However, this is not a quick undertaking, and fat is not the primary energy source. Furthermore, fat is not a good energy source for the brain. So, what happens if you limit carbohydrates for a prolonged period of time?

In the absence of carbohydrates, your liver synthesizes ketones from fats and provides a faster, more consistent supply of energy to your brain and organs. This ketogenesis phenomenon occurs when you follow a ketogenic diet. When ketogenesis kicks in, you enter ketosis.

What Are Ketones?

Ketosis is a hallmark of the ketogenic diet, but ketones are not. Ketones are naturally produced through fasting or strenuous activities. A keto diet causes ketone levels to be sustained and elevated, supplying energy to your body and brain, unlike any other diet.

After fasting for a night, ketones provide 6% energy but increase to 30 to 40% after three days and reach 60% or more during ketosis (Satrazemis, 2018).

Ketone bodies are made by your liver in three different forms:

- Acetoacetate
- Beta-hydroxybutyrate (BHB)
- Acetone

Acetoacetate is the primary ketone released by the liver when fatty acids are broken down or when carbohydrates are limited. It's then metabolized into BHB or acetone. Some acetoacetate is used as an energy source, and any surplus is passed through urination. BHB provides energy to your body when you are in ketosis. It also provides energy to your brain in a glucose-free environment. Ketosis is primarily about increasing BHB levels. Acetone has a lower reactivity than other ketones, making it the least significant ketone and is rarely produced. Since acetone leaves the body through exhalation, this is what causes "keto breath."

Get Into Ketosis in No Time

The following tips can help you achieve ketosis quickly while on a keto diet.

Reduce Carbs

Limiting carbohydrate intake is the most popular method of entering ketosis and maintaining it (Khan, 2016). However, the amount of carbohydrates needed to induce ketosis varies greatly—it falls anywhere between 20 grams to 70–100 grams for very athletic people.

A rough guideline is that approximately 5% of your daily calories should be derived from carbohydrates or about 20 grams of carbohydrates daily. If you need more calories or exercise a lot, I recommend starting with 50 grams of carbohydrates.

Increase Fat Consumption

Eating more fat by itself won't lead to ketosis. You can fuel your body by including more fat in your diet so that it can create ketones and support your metabolism. If you want to know how much fat you should consume on a ketogenic diet, you should check out one of the dozens of keto apps.

Eat Your MCTs

Plant-based fats are considered a good source of fat and are recommended in any diet, especially keto. However, in ketosis, saturated fats such as medium-chain triglycerides (MCTs) may be helpful. MCTs derived from saturated plant fats include palm and coconut oil and grass-fed dairy items like milk, cheese, and butter. MCT oil supplements are also available.

Exogenous Ketones Supplements

Ketone supplements may help you enter ketosis and stay in ketosis without eating a keto diet (Walle, 2018). Combined with MCTs, keto supplements may be beneficial. Of course, they cannot act as a replacement for a ketogenic diet.

Consider Intermittent Fasting

A 3-day fast can also help you enter ketosis faster. This method is not only challenging but difficult to maintain. Intermittent fasting or fasting for shorter periods of time is a good way to induce ketosis rapidly and maximize the effects of a ketogenic diet (Kubala, 2018). Be sure to verify the safety behind this long of a fast with a medical professional or primary doctor.

Approximately When Does the Body Go Into Ketosis?

Ketosis can occur at varying rates depending on your level of exercise, body composition, and overall nutrition. A day of carbohydrate restriction won't make a difference. Sugar has been your body's primary fuel source for years, and it takes time to adapt. Depletion of carbohydrate reserves is necessary to begin the process of fat burning. When a fit person begins a ketogenic diet, glycogen is burned within two days. Considering everything, getting into ketosis usually takes approximately 1–7 days.

Maintaining Ketosis

Staying in ketosis is as simple as remaining committed to your keto diet and eating low-carb foods. Track your macros with an app, and don't cheat too much! Getting into ketosis is as easy as one, two, three.

Chapter 4: What to Eat on a Ketogenic Diet?

What to Eat on a Ketogenic Diet?

What foods are allowed on a keto diet? Keep your beloved items close to your heart, but also branch out—going keto can really expand your palate as well as slim you down. Here is a list of healthy, keto-friendly foods to stock up on. Each one is delicious and catered to different tastes!

Keto-Friendly Foods

Vegetables
Greens (lettuce, arugula, kale, collards, chard, and rutabaga), shiitake, onion, chives, asparagus, mushrooms, avocado, eggplant, cauliflower, carrots, bok choy, radishes, tomatoes, broccoli, zucchini, and radishes.

In moderation: broccolini, cabbage, brussels sprouts, cauliflower, cabbage, green beans, fennel, snap peas, okra, fennel, and snow peas.

Fruits
Strawberries, blueberries, blackberries, oranges, lime, coconut, and lemons.

Ground Meat
Chicken, pork, beef, and turkey.

Lunch and Deli Meats
Bacon, pork slab, pepperoni, salami, bratwurst, chorizo, turkey, ham, kielbasa, pastrami, bacon, and sauerkraut.
In moderation: bologna and capicola.

Meat and Poultry

Beef, veal, duck, chicken, pork, lamb, turkey, and game.

Seafood

Fatty fish, white fish, oysters, octopus, prawns, scallops, clams, snails, lobsters, and crabs.

Dairy

Brie, blue cheese, parmesan, cheddar, provolone, mozzarella, gouda, cream cheese, goat, gruyere, and camembert; double cream, heavy cream, butter; eggs and ghee.

In moderation: milk, feta, pepper jack, crème fraîche, mascarpone, cottage cheese, sour cream, and ricotta.

Fats and Oils

Avocado oil, coconut oil, flaxseed oil, olive oil, cocoa butter, and peanut oil.

Schmaltz, duck fat, and lard.

Nuts and Seeds

Almonds, peanuts, brazil nuts, pecans, walnuts, macadamia, hazelnuts, chia seeds, pine nuts, pumpkin seeds, hemp seeds, sesame seeds, and flax seeds.

Keto-Friendly Drink Options

Tea, diet soda, coffee, sparkling water, seltzer, energy drinks (no carbs), and keto-approved smoothies.

Sauces and Dressings

Mustard, mayo, no sugar ketchup, vinegar, and hot sauce (be careful to read the nutritional information).

Canned Food

Crab, anchovies, tuna, salmon, tomato, sardines, pickles, olives, and sauerkraut (be careful to read the nutritional information).

Herbs and Spices

Dried or fresh and bouillon cubes.

Nut and Seed Butters

Almond butter, hazelnut butter, peanut butter, coconut butter, pecan butter, macadamia butter, walnut butter, sunflower seed butter, and tahini.

Baking Ingredients

Coconut flour, almond flour, baking powder, cocoa, baking soda, dark chocolate, vanilla extract, and glutamine powder.

Keto-Friendly Alcohol

Vodka, dry martini, whisky, tequila, and brandy.

In moderation: wine.

Vegetarian

Tofu, tempeh, jackfruit, shirataki noodles, full-fat coconut milk, nutritional yeast, kelp noodles, nori sheets, roasted seaweed, and kelp flakes.

Keto Sweeteners

Erythritol, stevia drops, Splenda, monk fruit, and xylitol.

Non-Keto-Friendly Foods

Grains

Wheat, quinoa, rice, oats, barley, corn, amaranth, millet, and buckwheat.

Starches

Sweet potatoes, beans, lentils, cassava, taro, plantain, banana, and mestizo.

Flours

Wheat flour, maize, arrowroot, potato starch, cassava, chickpeas, and fava beans.

Oils From Processed Vegetables and Trans Fats

Corn syrup, margarine, vegetable shortening, shortening, palm oil, rapeseed oil, linseed oil, grapeseed oil, vegetable oil, and soybean oil.

Sugars

Sugar and sweeteners of all types (sorghum syrup, malt syrup, rice syrup, high maltose corn syrup, carob syrup, and corn syrup), cane juice, cane juice crystals, barley malt, muscovado, malt, treacle, agave nectar, scant, panocha, maple syrup, honey, and molasses.

Farm-Raised Fish, Eggs, and Any Processed Meat

Low-Fat dairy

Fat-free butter, low-fat yogurts, evaporated skim milk, and reduced-fat cheese.

Sugary drinks

Soda.

Fruits

All fruits, including dried, except for berries

Chapter 5: Maintaining a Macronutrient Ratio

Macronutrients, or 'macros,' include carbohydrates, fats, and proteins, and they encompass nutrients that are energy-rich. Keto macros can be calculated online in a matter of minutes with a keto app. You can use it to determine how much macronutrients to consume if you are trying to lose or maintain.

Fats

A ketogenic diet must include fats. You must choose the right fats on a keto diet as some fats are more weight-loss-friendly and nutritious. Fat is what burns fat. Avoiding fat and eating a lot of proteins, such as poultry and seafood, will convert excess protein into glucose. This will also increase insulin production.

Remember that your body requires a variety of fats, namely saturated and unsaturated fats. Unsaturated fats are divided into two categories:

- polyunsaturated fats (omega-3 and omega-6)
- monounsaturated fats

Monounsaturated fatty acids can be found in oils made from peanuts, canola, sesame seeds, cocoa, and walnuts. Polyunsaturated fats are found in seeds, fatty fish, soybean oil, and nuts. Saturated fats are found in cheese, butter, beef, cream, and poultry with skin, pork, and lard. Trans fats are processed unsaturated fats. Reduce your intake of saturated and trans fats to prevent cardiovascular disease, hypertension, and diabetes.

Packaged foods and fast food contain high levels of saturated fat. As a result, you should limit sweets and snacks like doughnuts; takeaway; high-fat fast food like french fries, pizza, and burgers; and sweets like cake and cookies.

Protein

Proteins also play an essential part in human health. It is made up of smaller molecules known as amino acids, and you need them to survive. Proteins play a number of important roles, such as producing hormones, regulating weight, maintaining health, developing muscle, and healing the body. Protein is essential for skin, skeletal, and mental development. On a keto diet, protein-rich foods include fish, beef, chicken, cheese, and eggs. Nuts and seeds are good sources of plant protein.

Carbohydrates

We convert carbohydrates into glucose. Organs like the liver, brain, and kidneys require carbohydrates to work effectively. An excessive intake of carbs, however, causes fat to accumulate.

Micronutrients

Micronutrients are also necessary for survival, and they include vitamins and minerals. It is important to remember that most micronutrients and phytonutrients are concentrated in vegetables and, therefore, keto veggies should be a part of each meal. Knowing your macros, a ketogenic diet can be planned with ease. My simple 7-day meal plan can help you get started.

Chapter 6: 7-Day Keto Meal Plan for Beginners

I created a simple meal plan to help you start your keto lifestyle. By following this 7-day keto meal plan, you can enjoy the benefits of eating low-carb meals without the hassle and anxiety of making decisions at a moment's notice.

Day 1

Breakfast: 1 tbsp of almond butter; 1 slice of cauliflower bread

Lunch: Citrus Avocado Shrimp Salad

Dinner: Pepper Steak Stir-Fry

Day 2

Breakfast: 1 hard-boiled egg; 2 slices of bacon; ½ an avocado

Lunch: Grilled Chicken Cobb Salad

Dinner: Yummy Coconut Pork Chops

Day 3

Breakfast: Green Goddess Smoothie; 10 Almonds

Lunch: Salmon Rolls

Dinner: Pan-Seared Sea Bass

Day 4

Breakfast: 2 boiled eggs; 1 slice of bacon; cauliflower bread

Lunch: Citrus Avocado Shrimp Salad

Dinner: Pepper Steak Stir-Fry

Day 5

Breakfast: Savory Chicken Muffins

Lunch: Grilled Chicken Cobb Salad

Dinner: Easy Keto Chicken Chili

Day 6

Breakfast: Green Goddess Smoothie

Lunch: Salmon Rolls

Dinner: Pan-Seared Sea Bass

Day 7

Breakfast: 1 hard-boiled egg; 2 slices of bacon; ½ an avocado

Lunch: Savory Chicken Muffins

Dinner: Yummy Coconut Pork Chops

Recipes

Cauliflower Bread

I love this recipe for cauliflower bread. Sandwiches, toast, and any bread-based meal can be substituted with it.

Time: 35 minutes

Serving Size: 6 servings

Prep Time: 10 minutes

Cook Time: 25 minutes

Nutritional Facts/Info:

Calories: 200 cal

Carbs: 9 g

Fat: 3 g

Protein: 7 g

Ingredients:

- 1 tsp olive oil
- 1 small onion
- 1 finely minced cauliflower head
- 1 cup chopped spinach

- ½ cup chopped almonds
- 3 whisked eggs
- 2 minced garlic cloves
- 1 tbsp fresh oregano
- A pinch of salt and black pepper

Directions:

1. Over medium heat, warm up the oil and add the onion. Mix them and sauté for 10 minutes.
2. Add in the spinach, almonds, cauliflower, garlic, oregano, eggs, salt, and pepper. Mix the ingredients together, place them in a loaf pan, and bake at 350 °F for 15 minutes.
3. Cut into even slices and enjoy your breakfast.

Green Goddess Smoothie

The green goddess smoothie is filled with antioxidants, vitamins, and fats that will help you feel full between meals. Healthy and delicious, it makes the perfect keto breakfast.

Time: 5 minutes

Serving Size: 6 servings

Prep Time: 5 minutes

Cook Time: 0 minutes

Nutritional Facts/Info:

Calories: 200 cal

Carbs: 9 g

Fat: 2 g

Protein: 5 g

Ingredients:

- 4 cups water
- 1/3 cup frozen strawberry slices
- 1 cup baby spinach, shredded
- 2 tbsp hemp seeds
- 1 tbsp ginger, minced
- 1 cup cucumber, sliced
- ½ cup kiwi, skinned
- ½ cup frozen avocado chunks

Directions:

1. In a blender, combine the water, baby spinach, strawberries, hemp seeds, ginger, cucumber, avocado, and kiwi. Mix well, pour into glasses, and enjoy.

Savory Chicken Muffins

I've got the perfect high-protein chicken muffin recipe for you that's perfect for meal prepping! These Savory Chicken Muffins are packed with protein, made with basic ingredients, and the ultimate breakfast treat.

Time: 1 hour 10 minutes

Serving Size: 3 servings

Prep Time: 10 minutes

Cook Time: 1 hour

Nutritional Facts/Info:

Calories: 270 cal

Carbs: 16 g

Fat: 5 g

Protein: 10 g

Ingredients:

- 1 lb chicken breast, skinless and without bone (or any cooked protein)
- A dash of salt and black pepper
- ½ tsp garlic powder
- 2 tbsp bacon bits
- 3 tbsp hot sauce
- 6 eggs
- 2 tbsp coconut oil, heated
- 2 tbsp green onions, chopped
- ¼ cup cheddar cheese

Directions:

1. Place the chicken breasts on a baking sheet, sprinkle with salt and pepper, and bake at 425 °F for 25 minutes.
2. Shred the meat with two forks, place it in a bowl, and add the cheese, bacon bits, hot sauce, and ghee. Toss well.
3. Using a separate bowl, combine the eggs with pepper, salt, and green onions.
4. Divide the egg mixture among six muffin cups. Add the meat and bake at 425 °F for 30 minutes.

Citrus Avocado Shrimp Salad

Citrus Avocado Shrimp Salad is a delicious dish that doesn't require much preparation. The combination of lime and cilantro creates a delightful, nutritious salad that you'll want to eat again and again.

Time: 15 minutes

Serving Size: 2 servings

Prep Time: 10 minutes

Cook Time: 5 minutes

Nutritional Facts/Info:

Calories: 320 cal

Carbs: 15 g

Fat: 15 g

Protein: 6 g

Ingredients:

- 1 avocado, skinned and diced
- 8 oz jumbo cooked, peeled shrimp, chopped
- 1/3 cup feta cheese, grated
- 1 tomato, diced
- ¼ cup cilantro, chopped
- 2 tbsp ghee
- 1 tbsp olive oil
- 1 tbsp lime juice
- A dash of salt and black pepper

Directions:

1. Toss the shrimp with the ghee in a bowl.
2. Preheat a pan over medium-high heat, add in the shrimp, and sear them for 5 minutes, Then, remove them to a bowl.
3. Add avocado, lemon juice, tomato, cheese, oil, salt, pepper, and parsley. Combine all together and enjoy.

Grilled Chicken Cobb Salad

This Grilled Chicken Cobb Salad combines the classic flavors of the original salad with a keto-friendly dressing. Made with cherry tomatoes, lettuce, cucumber, bacon, cheese, and avocado, it's delicious for a lunch or picnic!

Time: 45 minutes

Serving Size: 4 servings

Prep Time: 35 minutes

Cook Time: 10 minutes

Nutritional Facts/Info:

Calories: 300 cal

Carbs: 10 g

Fat: 15 g

Protein: 10 g

Ingredients:

- 2 tbsp olive oil
- ¼ cup lemon juice
- 2 tbsp red vinegar
- 2 tbsp water
- 2 tsp garlic, minced
- 2 tsp basil, dried
- 1 tsp oregano, dried
- 1 lb boneless skinless chicken breasts, pounded to even thickness
- 4 cups mixed green lettuce leaves
- 3 hard-boiled eggs
- 6 slices of bacon cooked and chopped
- 1 red onion, diced
- 1 cucumber, diced
- 1 cup cherry tomatoes, halved
- 1 avocado, diced
- ½ cup crumbled blue cheese

For the vinaigrette:

- 4 tbsp apple cider vinegar
- 2 tbsp sour cream
- ½ tsp garlic powder
- 2 tbsp extra virgin olive oil
- Pinch of salt and pepper to taste

Directions:

1. In a large bowl, mix the chicken with 1 tbsp of oil, vinegar, lemon juice, parsley, water, garlic, oregano, and basil. Mix well and chill for 30 minutes.

2. In a medium pot, place the eggs and pour them over with water.
3. Put the pot on high heat and cover it with a lid. Let the water boil.
4. Once the water reaches a boil, turn off the heat and let the eggs rest for 15 minutes, covered. Place eggs in a large bowl of icy water and run cold water over them until the water is cool. Let the eggs sit in the chilled water for about 8–10 minutes. When they are cool, remove the shells and slice them.
5. On medium-high heat, warm up the remaining oil in your kitchen grill. Place the chicken and grill them for 5 minutes on each side. Remove them from the pan and onto a plate. Slice, and arrange on a plate.
6. Mix all the ingredients for the vinaigrette together. Drizzle 1 tsp on top of the avocado slices to prevent oxidation.
7. Add bacon, lettuce, onion, tomatoes, cucumber, avocado, cheese, and more of the marinade. Combine and enjoy.

Salmon Nori Sushi Roll

With this easy recipe, you can indulge in keto sushi at home using nori seaweed sheets, cucumber, salmon, red peppers, and avocado. They are healthy, guilt-free, and delicious. Sushi for everyone!

Time: 10 minutes

Serving Size: 3 servings

Prep Time: 10 minutes

Cook Time: 0 minutes

Nutritional Facts/Info:

Calories: 200 cal

Carbs: 11 g

Fat: 4 g

Protein: 5 g

Ingredients:

- 3 nori sheets
- 5 oz cooked salmon or tinned salmon
- 1 red pepper, thinly sliced
- 1 small avocado, thinly sliced
- 1 small cucumber, thinly sliced
- 1 spring onion, chopped into 2–3" slices
- 1 tbsp mayonnaise
- Coconut aminos for serving, optional

Directions:

1. On a cutting board, lay out the nori sheets. Assemble the salmon, cucumber, mayonnaise, bell pepper, avocado, and onion on the nori sheets. Each roll should be cut into two pieces and served with coconut aminos.

Keto Chicken Chili

You might be inspired to whip up your favorite batch of chili. However, not all chili recipes are keto-friendly. Try this simple keto chicken chili recipe to spice things up!

Time: 1 hour 30 minutes

Serving Size: 6 servings

Prep Time: 10 minutes

Cook Time: 20 minutes

Nutritional Facts/Info:

Calories: 220 cal

Carbs: 15 g

Fat: 5 g

Protein: 10 g

Ingredients:

- 1 lb chicken, minced
- 2 garlic cloves, crushed
- 1 onion, diced
- 1 and ½ tbsp avocado oil
- 1 tbsp chili powder
- 3 chili peppers, seeded and diced finely
- 28 oz canned tomatoes, diced
- 3 cups butternut squash, peeled and diced
- 14 oz chicken stock
- A dash of salt and black pepper

Directions:

1. Warm up the oil in a pot over medium-high heat. Add in onion, chicken, and garlic, and cook for six minutes, stirring occasionally.
2. Add chili powder, stock, chilies, squash, tomatoes, salt, and pepper. Mix together, cover it, and cook for 15 minutes. Serve.

Pan-Seared Sea Bass

A delicious seafood dinner of Pan-seared Sea Bass is only minutes away. The sea bass shows off its star quality with just the right amount of seasoning.

Time: 25 minutes

Serving Size: 2 servings

Prep Time: 10 minutes

Cook Time: 15 minutes

Nutritional Facts/Info:

Calories: 320 cal

Carbs: 9 g

Fat: 6 g

Protein: 20 g

Ingredients:

- 2 sea bass filets, boneless and skinless
- 1 orange, peeled and sliced
- 1 broccoli head, divided into florets
- A pinch of salt and black pepper
- 3 tbsp olive oil (extra virgin)
- 4 tbsp capers
- Wedged lemons (optional garnish)

Directions:

1. Over medium-high heat, add two tablespoons of oil and sea bass filets. Sprinkle with salt and pepper, and sear for four minutes on the skin side. Flip, cook for two minutes more, and divide.
2. In another pan, warm up the remaining oil over medium-high heat. Add capers, broccoli, orange, pepper, and salt. Mix and cook for six minutes.
3. Remove from the pan. Add a squeeze of fresh lemon juice, and serve!

Pepper Steak Stir-Fry

The best keto-friendly dinner is a simple meat and vegetable meal. Pepper Steak Stir-Fry has always been a go-to meal of mine. It's great for busy weeknights since it takes no more than 25 minutes to prepare. It's even quicker if all the ingredients are prepped and ready.

Time: 25 minutes

Serving Size: 4 servings

Prep Time: 10 minutes

Cook Time: 15 minutes

Nutritional Facts/Info:

Calories: 300 cal

Carbs: 15 g

Fat: 4 g

Protein: 22 g

Ingredients:

- 1 tbsp avocado oil
- 1 onion, chopped
- 1 medium bell pepper sliced into ribbons
- 1 garlic clove
- 1 lb sirloin or flank steak sliced into thin slices
- ½ cup beef broth
- 2 tbsp soy sauce or tamari
- 8 oz mushrooms sliced
- A pinch of salt and black pepper

Directions:

1. Warm up the oil in a pan over medium-high heat, then add the onions. Mix and cook for 3 minutes.
2. Brown the beef strips and garlic in the oil. Once the beef is cooked, season with salt and pepper, and remove from the pan.
3. If necessary, add more oil. Cook onion and pepper in a pan until soft.
4. Add in the mushrooms, broth, and soy sauce. Simmer for a few minutes until soft.
5. Stir in the beef and cook until heated through.

Yummy Coconut Pork Chops

The golden, tender, and succulent pork chops are smothered in a delicious creamy coconut-garlic mushroom sauce bursting with flavor. The recipe is simple and takes only 40 minutes to prepare.

Time: 40 minutes

Serving Size: 4 servings

Prep Time: 10 minutes

Cook Time: 30 minutes

Nutritional Facts/Info:

Calories: 330 cal

Carbs: 12 g

Fat: 8 g

Protein: 11 g

Ingredients:

- 3 bacon slices, chopped
- 4 cloves garlic, crushed
- 1 tbsp olive oil
- 1 small onion, diced
- 8 oz mushrooms, sliced
- 4 pork chops, bone-in or boneless (about 1-inch thick)
- 1 cup veggie stock
- ½ oz oregano, sliced
- 10 oz coconut cream
- 1 tbsp parsley, minced

Directions:

1. Warm up the oil in a skillet over medium-high heat. Add the bacon and cook for two minutes.

2. Add in the mushroom, garlic, and onion, and cook for three minutes.
3. Add the pork chops, stock, oregano, and garlic powder, and bring to a simmer. Cook for 30 minutes.
4. Pour in the coconut cream and parsley. Mix and cook for another 10 minutes. Serve.

Conclusion

The foundation of success in life is good health: that is the substratum fortune; it is also the basis of happiness. A person cannot accumulate a fortune very well when he is sick. -P. T. Barnum

I hope you have enjoyed reading this book and that the information and knowledge you have gained helps you reap the ketogenic benefits.

Most people who stand to gain from a low-carb, moderate-protein, high-fat, ketogenic diet don't even consider it. I find that to be the greatest tragedy. Approximately what percentage of your loved ones suffer from a condition that could be aided by the keto diet—type 2 diabetes, hypertension, epilepsy, heart disease, Alzheimer's, menopause, and countless others? Isn't it time they learned about a safe dietary treatment that might supplement medications and outperform other approaches? Absolutely! This book was driven by my desire to provide straightforward, easy-to-understand details about ketosis and the keto diet. My goal was to equip you with the information, understanding, and confidence to pursue the keto diet to improve your overall health.

Making simple lifestyle changes is the secret to success. Follow the 7-day ketogenic meal plan provided; stick to simple dishes like salads and stews. Choose simple snacks as well. Clean out and organize your kitchen, and prepare easy meals. Relax, breathe, and enjoy the fresh air. Being outdoors and enjoying life with loved ones makes it easier to maintain a healthy diet.

Now it's your turn. People around you, friends, and family may be curious about your actions. You should now be able to walk around as a living, thriving example of what you can achieve when you try the keto diet. It's time to get cooking!

Glossary

Electrolytes: Electrolytes are electrochemically charged minerals in the body that are necessary for proper cellular function. Whenever you begin a brand-new diet, your fluid content as well as your electrolyte balance changes. On the keto diet, replenishing electrolytes is essential.

Erythritol: A sugar alcohol that is an organic sugar substitute with no calories. If possible, use a GMO-free variety.

Exogenous Ketones: Ketone bodies that are taken as supplements. Exogenous ketones help people accelerate ketosis and reduce keto flu discomfort. However, they shouldn't be used indefinitely.

Himalayan Pink Salt: Most minerals in table salt have been removed. Himalayan pink salt is handy when starting a keto diet because it flushes electrolytes out of the body.

Intermittent Fasting: During this type of fast, a person cycles between fasting and consuming food.

Keto: Keto refers to the ketogenic diet. When people talk about the keto diet or refer to it as the keto diet, they are alluding to the ketogenic diet. The ketogenic diet is designed to force your body to stop utilizing carbs—glucose—as its primary energy and burn fat—ketones).

Keto Flu: A condition that occurs when the body adjusts to ketosis and the keto diet. While some people find this stressful, others might only encounter favorable effects, such as an energy boost or a slimmer figure.

Ketones: As the body quits burning glucose for energy, it starts burning fat for energy instead.

Ketosis: Ketosis is a state in which the body produces more ketones. Ketosis is the aim of the keto diet. The body burns fat for energy rather than carbs if ketones are elevated.

Macros or Macronutrients: These are nutrients we require in large amounts to live. They are carbohydrates, fats, proteins, and water. A ketogenic diet usually comprises 60–75% fats, 15–30% protein, and 5–10% carbohydrates.

Net Carbs: When counting macros, there are several ways to calculate carbs. You can count total carbohydrates or net carbohydrates. To calculate net carbohydrates, subtract fiber from total carbohydrates. Fibrous foods are not absorbed in the small intestine, so they don't have the same effect as sugar.

Stevia: Organic sugar substitute derived from stevia plants. It has very few calories.

References

Boden, G., Sargrad, K., Homko, C., Mozzoli, M., & Stein, T. P. (2005, March 15). Effect of a low-carbohydrate diet on appetite, blood glucose levels, and insulin resistance in obese patients with type 2 diabetes. *Annals of Internal Medicine, 142*(6), 403. https://doi.org/10.7326/0003-4819-142-6-200503150-00006

Eldridge, L. (2022, June 10). *Ketogenic diet and cancer.* Verywell Health. https://www.verywellhealth.com/ketogenic-diet-and-cancer-4773058

Khan, N. (2016, November 21). *7 Effective Tips to Get Into Ketosis.* Healthline. https://www.healthline.com/nutrition/7-tips-to-get-into-ketosis

Kubala, J. (2018, November 5). *Intermittent fasting and keto: Should you combine the two?* Healthline. https://www.healthline.com/nutrition/intermittent-fasting-and-keto

Licquia, A. (2017, April 28). Ketogenic Diet. Kadlec Tri-Cities Cancer Center. https://tccancer.org/news/ketogenic-diet-anyway/#:~:text=The%20Ketogenic%20Diet%20was%20designed

Mawer, R. (2020, October 22). *The ketogenic diet: A detailed beginner's guide to keto.* Healthline. https://www.healthline.com/nutrition/ketogenic-diet-101#:~:text=Keto%20basics

Satrazemis, E. (2018, October 23). *How to get into ketosis: 6 steps backed by science.* Trifecta. https://www.trifectanutrition.com/blog/how-to-get-into-ketosis-tips-backed-by-science

Sullivan, M. G. (2021, June 7). *Can a ketogenic diet reduce Alzheimer's risks and symptoms?* AARP. https://www.aarp.org/health/dementia/info-2021/keto-diet-alzheimers.html

Walle, G. V. D. (2018, October 23). *Do exogenous ketone supplements work for weight loss?* Healthline.

Printed in Great Britain
by Amazon

86881877R00027